D0554897

Medicine in Colonial America

Charlie Samuel

The Rosen Publishing Group's
PowerKids Press™
New York

Published in 2003 by The Rosen Publishing Group, Inc.
29 East 21st Street, New York, NY 10010

First Edition

Photo Credits: Key: t:top; b:below; c: center; l: left; r: right
p.5tr AKG London; pp.5cl, 7tl Corbis/Bettmann; p.8 AKG London pp.7b, 8br, 11bl Peter Newark's American Pictures; p.11cr Werner Forman Archive/National Museum of Denmark; p.12tl & cr Peter Newark's American Pictures; p.12bl Corbis/Bettmann; p.15t Peter Newark's American Pictures; p.15b Bridgeman Art Library; p.16 Science & Society Picture Library; p. 20tr Peter Newark's American Pictures; p.20bl Corbis/Bettmann.

Library of Congress Cataloging-in-Publication Data

Samuel, Charlie.
   Medicine in colonial America / Charlie Samuel.
      v. cm. – (Primary sources of everyday life in colonial America)
Includes bibliographical references and index.
Contents: The New World – The difficult trip to North America – Native Americans face European diseases – Native American medicine – Colonial doctors and hospitals – Benjamin Rush – Inside an apothecary's shop – Medical supplies – Smallpox – Beyond colonial medicine.
   ISBN 0-8239-6598-8
   1. Medicine–United States–History–17th century. 2.Medicine–United States–History–18th century. [1. Medicine–United States–History–17th century. 2. Medicine–United States–History–18th century.] I. Title. II. Series.
   E188 .S19 2003
   610'.973'09032–dc21
                                                    2002004486

Contents

1. The New World 5

2. The Difficult Trip to North America 6

3. Native Americans Face European
   Diseases 9

4. Native American Medicine 10

5. Disease in Colonial Communities 13

6. Medical Practices 14

7. Medical Supplies 17

8. Inside an Apothecary's Shop 18

9. Benjamin Rush 20

10. Beyond Colonial Medicine 22

Glossary 23

Index 24

Primary Sources............................. 24

Web Sites..................................... 24

► Louis XIV, King of France, sent some of his subjects to America. He wanted France's colonies to be more powerful than England's colonies.

▼ The English government encouraged people to settle in America using posters like this one.

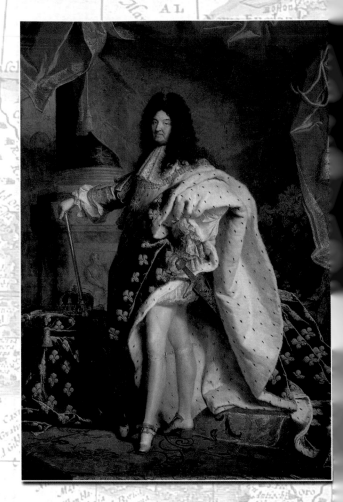

▼ Roanoke, settled in 1584, was the first English colony in America. The colonists soon all disappeared. No one knows what happened to them.

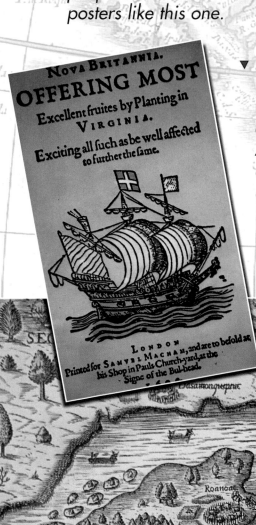

NOVA BRITANNIA.

OFFERING MOST

Excellent fruites by Planting in
VIRGINIA.

Exciting all such as be well affected
to further the same.

LONDON
Printed for SAMVEL MACHAM, and are to be fold at
his Shop in Pauls Church-yard, at the
Signe of the Bul-head.

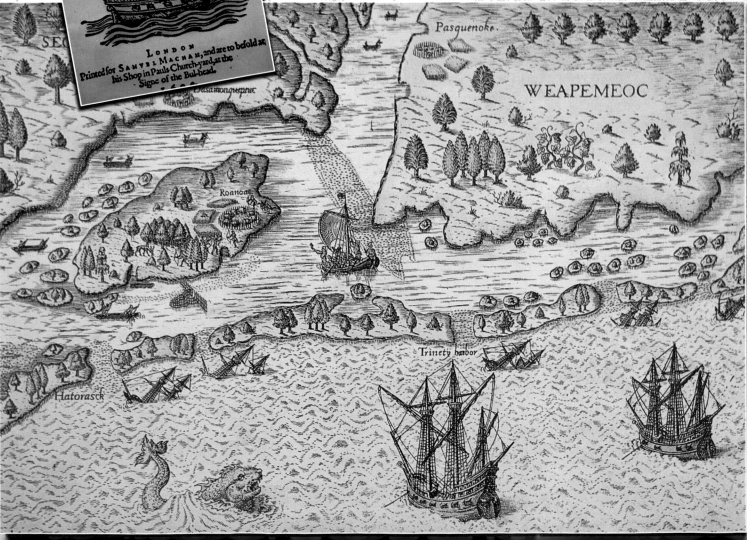

The New World

When Europeans heard about America just before 1500, they called it the New World, even though people already lived there. Stories said that America was rich in gold, fish, and furs. The soil was good for farming. The New World sounded like a good place to live.

The Spaniards soon set up **colonies** in Mexico and the American Southwest. France claimed colonies in present-day Canada, and later in the area west of the Mississippi River. England had 13 colonies. By 1669 the English claimed all the East Coast, from New England to Georgia.

The Europeans soon found that the New World was not like Europe. It had animals they did not recognize. Their crops would not grow in the soil. They went hungry. They got sick.

There were no hospitals. Doctors did not know that **diseases** spread through **germs** too small to see. Disease spread rapidly among the settlers and the Native Americans they met.

The Difficult Trip to North America

Many settlers did not even reach America. The journey from Europe could take as long as four months. The seas could be stormy. There was little fresh food on the ships. Diseases such as **scurvy** were common. At the end of 1606, 144 men left England to begin the colony of Virginia. Only 100 survived the journey to America.

The English colonists soon started to bring enslaved African people to the colonies. They made them work on large farms called **plantations**. The journey to America was even worse for slaves. They were packed close together. They did not have enough to eat. They had no medical care. If slaves got seriously ill, the slave traders threw them overboard.

Life was not easy for colonists who reached America. Some learned from Native Americans what crops to grow or what wild plants to eat. Others made enemies of native peoples. Many colonists died from either starvation or disease.

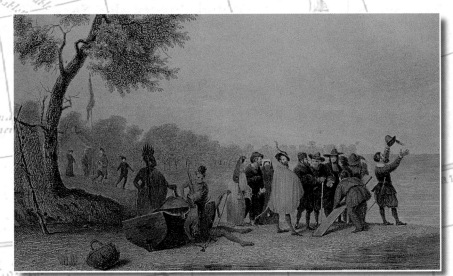

◄ The first settlers land at Jamestown in 1607. Within three years most of them were dead from either sickness or starvation.

▼ If a slave got sick on the way to America, the crew of the slave ship threw him or her into the sea to die.

▼ The Pilgrims prepare to sail to America onboard the Mayflower in 1620. Some of them died from sickness before they reached the New World.

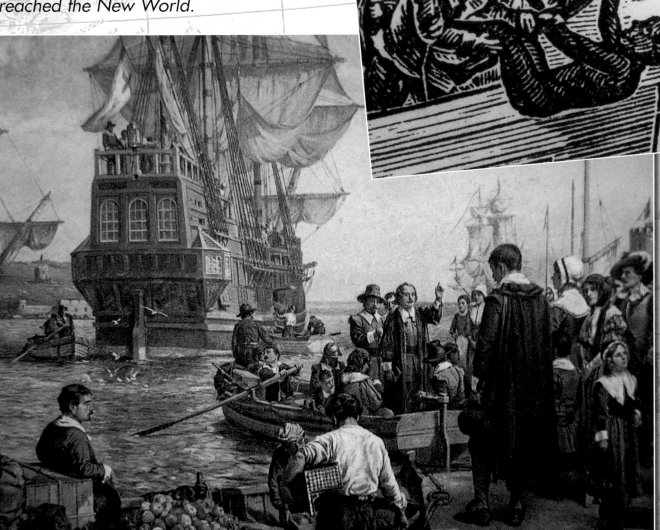

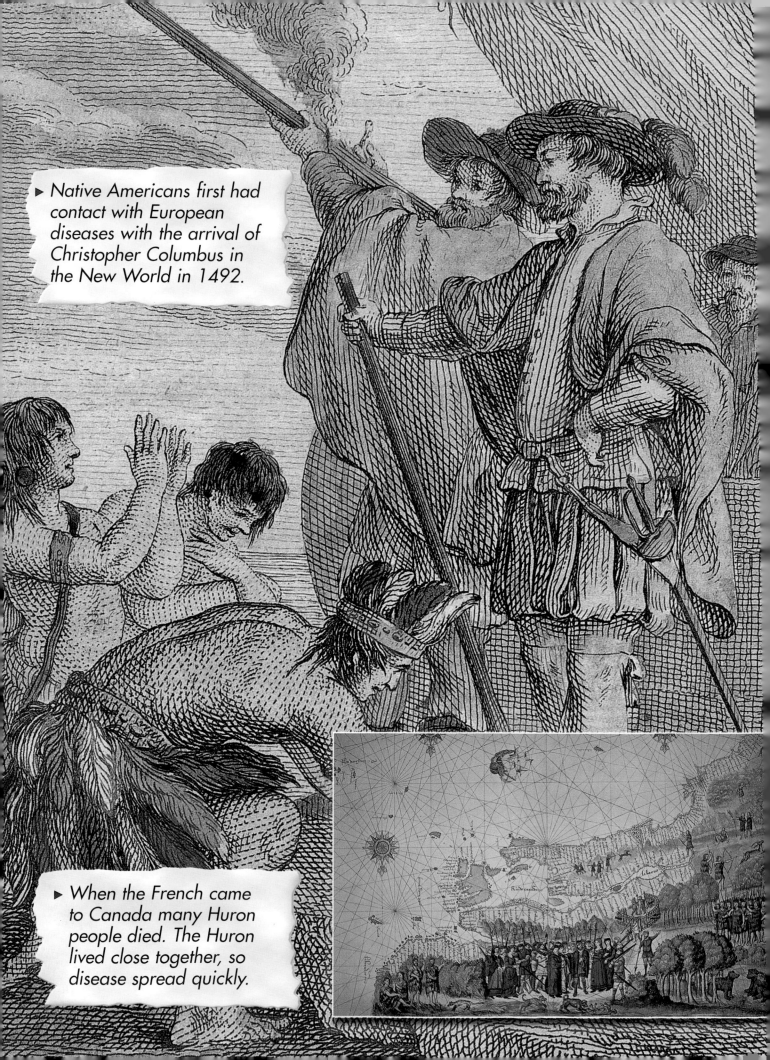

▶ Native Americans first had contact with European diseases with the arrival of Christopher Columbus in the New World in 1492.

▶ When the French came to Canada many Huron people died. The Huron lived close together, so disease spread quickly.

Native Americans Face European Diseases

The arrival of the Europeans brought death for millions of Native Americans. No one knew much about diseases or how they spread. They were carried by germs, which were too small to see. Europeans did not realize that they were carrying diseases because they did not always get sick themselves. If people are in contact with a disease over a long period, they can develop a resistance to it, called an **immunity**.

Native Americans had no immunity to serious European diseases such as measles, typhus, and smallpox. In Virginia smallpox killed one-third of all Native Americans in 60 years. When the Spaniards settled in Florida, 24 out of every 25 natives died within a century. Because they had no immunity, Native Americans could die from diseases, like colds, that were not serious for most Europeans. Diseases killed far more Native Americans than warfare did.

Native American Medicine

Over centuries Native Americans had learned how to make medicine from plants. Also, they moved from hot, damp places in summer to avoid insects that spread diseases through their bites. Because they washed every day, Native Americans were cleaner than the English.

Native Americans believed that sickness was caused by bad spirits. They asked the medicine man or woman, known as the **shaman**, to rid their bodies of these spirits. The shaman knew special rituals. He or she also knew good plants to clean diseases from the body. A paste made of flax helped treat pain in the body's joints, for example. The shaman made herbs and roots into drinks or into pastes. The sick also took **sweat baths**. Sweating helped get rid of fevers. However, it could not fight off serious diseases.

The English laughed at native medicine. They said it was based on magic. Even so, they tried to learn from the Native Americans about different ways to cure disease.

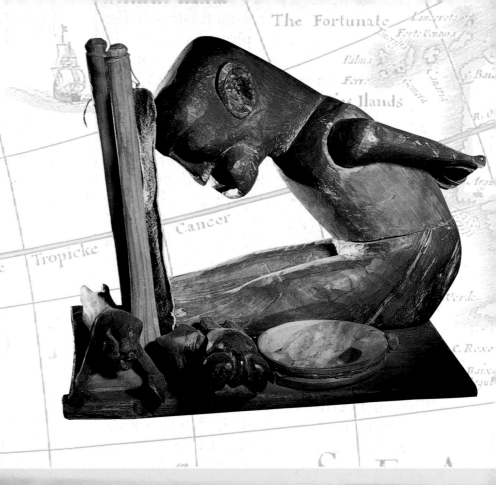

- This carving shows a shaman in a dreamlike state. The two animals are the spirits that help him.

▼ Shamans made medicine bundles, like this eagle tied up in cloth, to help cure diseases. They used the power of the animals from the spirit world.

▶▼ This Assiniboine man has just come out of a sweat bath, which is a small tent with a fire inside it. Sweating helped keep the skin clean.

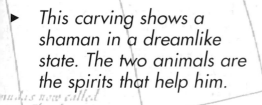

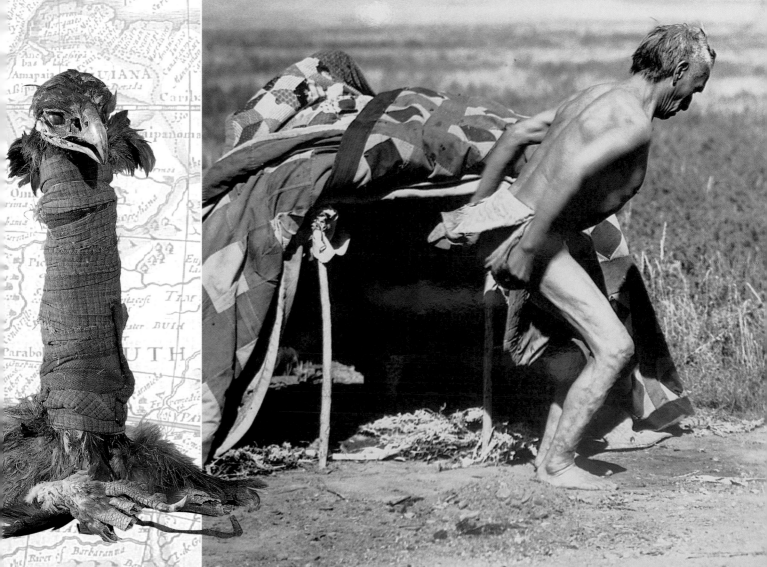

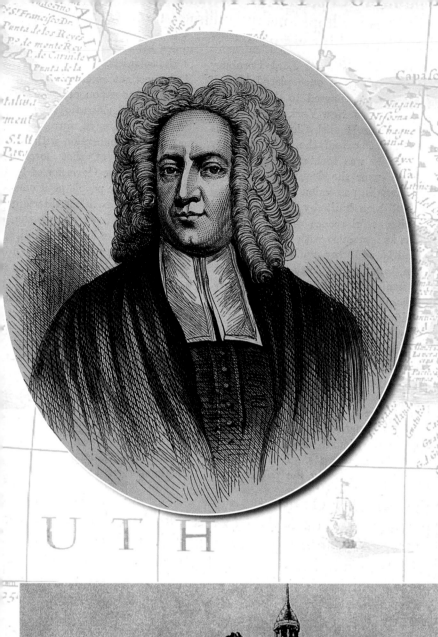

◄ Cotton Mather was a religious leader in New England at the end of the seventeenth century. He believed that inoculation against smallpox was a good idea, although some people thought it was dangerous.

▼ This notice about the sale of some slaves is careful to explain that they do not have smallpox or other diseases. No one wanted to buy a sick slave.

TO BE SOLD on board the Ship *Bance-Ifland*, on tuefday the 6th of *May* next, at *Afhley-Ferry*; a choice cargo of about 250 fine healthy

NEGROES,

juft arrived from the Windward & Rice Coaft.
—The utmoft care has already been taken, and fhall be continued, to keep them free from the leaft danger of being infected with the SMALL-POX, no boat having been on board, and all other communication with people from *Charles-Town* prevented.

Auftin, Laurens, & Appleby.

N. B. Full one Half of the above Negroes have had the SMALL-POX in their own Country.

BOSTON'S FIRST TOWN-HOUSE
1657–1711

◄ Colonial towns, like Boston, were dirty and very crowded. Disease spread easily among the population.

Disease in Colonial Communities

Communities were often crowded and dirty. There was little water for washing. There were no bathrooms. There was garbage in the street. Colonists often had **lice**, or small bugs, in their hair. **Vermin** like rats carried germs into houses.

The dirty conditions spread many kinds of sickness. Cuts and burns got **infected** very easily. Mosquitos carried diseases such as **malaria** and yellow fever. These diseases made people very sick or even killed them. When slave ships came from Africa they brought a new kind of malaria. It was even more deadly.

Two of the most feared diseases were bubonic plague and smallpox. The plague had killed millions of Europeans in the fourteenth century. It came to America soon after the first settlers. Smallpox, which killed many Native Americans, also killed colonists and slaves. Some of the colonists tried to prevent smallpox by a method called **inoculation**.

Medical Practices

People looked after anyone in their family who got sick. They had books that told them how to make creams and tonics for different diseases. Honeysuckle helped treat fevers and sore throats, for example. Cream made from foxglove plants helped to heal scabs. People also bought drugs from **merchants**.

There were few doctors and few hospitals. Colonial doctors did not study at a university. They learned by working with an older doctor for six years. Doctors' services were expensive and many people did not trust doctors. They preferred to use **midwives** or folk healers, who could make cures from plants. Barbers also often acted as doctors, even performing operations.

Having an operation was painful and dangerous. Surgeons' knives were blunt and their hands were dirty. They carried germs from one patient to another. There were no painkillers. Patients often died from either shock or infection. Many women died giving birth.

THE PACIFICKE

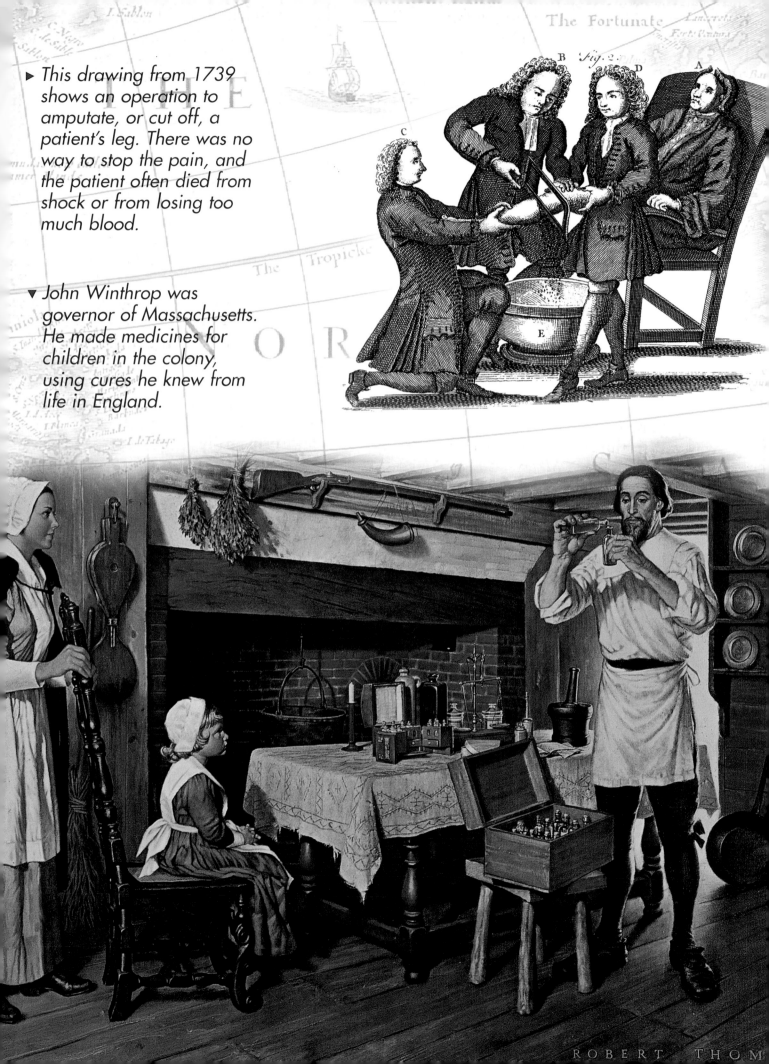

▶ This drawing from 1739 shows an operation to amputate, or cut off, a patient's leg. There was no way to stop the pain, and the patient often died from shock or from losing too much blood.

▼ John Winthrop was governor of Massachusetts. He made medicines for children in the colony, using cures he knew from life in England.

ROBERT THOM

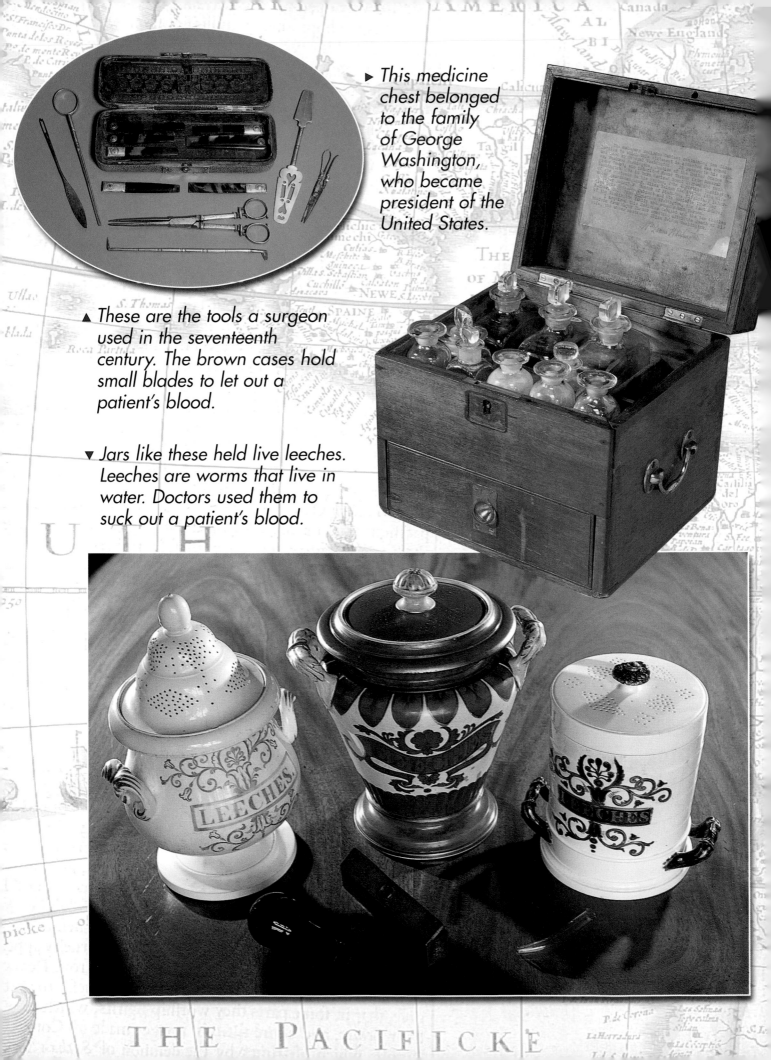

▶ This medicine chest belonged to the family of George Washington, who became president of the United States.

▲ These are the tools a surgeon used in the seventeenth century. The brown cases hold small blades to let out a patient's blood.

▼ Jars like these held live leeches. Leeches are worms that live in water. Doctors used them to suck out a patient's blood.

LEECHES

LEECHES

Medical Supplies

The colonists in America used many of the same cures that Europeans used. Some cures had been handed down in colonists' families. The colonists learned other cures from Native Americans. A paste made from cranberries helped wounds to heal quickly, for example. Parsley was good for soothing painful stomach aches. The leaves of a plant called columbine could be made into a lotion that would cure a sore throat or mouth. People grew plants in their gardens to make their own medicine. They kept the medicine in a wooden chest.

Doctors believed that sickness was caused by poison. They used medicine to make people throw up or go to the bathroom, which cleaned out the body. Another way they tried to get rid of disease was to remove some of a person's blood. The doctor cut the patient with sharp knives or used blood-sucking **leeches** to take out one or two pints of blood. If they took too much, the patient died.

Inside an Apothecary's Shop

The apothecary was like a druggist today. He made and sold medicines. Most medicines were made by mixing plants together. The apothecary gathered leaves, tree bark, and other materials from around the settlement. His store had many drawers in which to keep these supplies.

On the counter the apothecary kept a balance for weighing. It was important to use the right amount of each ingredient. Then he cut up the different plants with a knife and put them into a stone bowl called a mortar. He ground them into a powder with a small club called a pestle.

Once the apothecary had ground a powder he might store it in a glass jar until he needed to use it. He **dissolved** some powders in liquid to make a medicine that people could drink.

Making medicine was a slow business. The apothecary kept a stool in his shop where people sat while they waited for their cure.

▶ *This picture shows an apothecary using a pestle and mortar in his shop in the 1700s.*

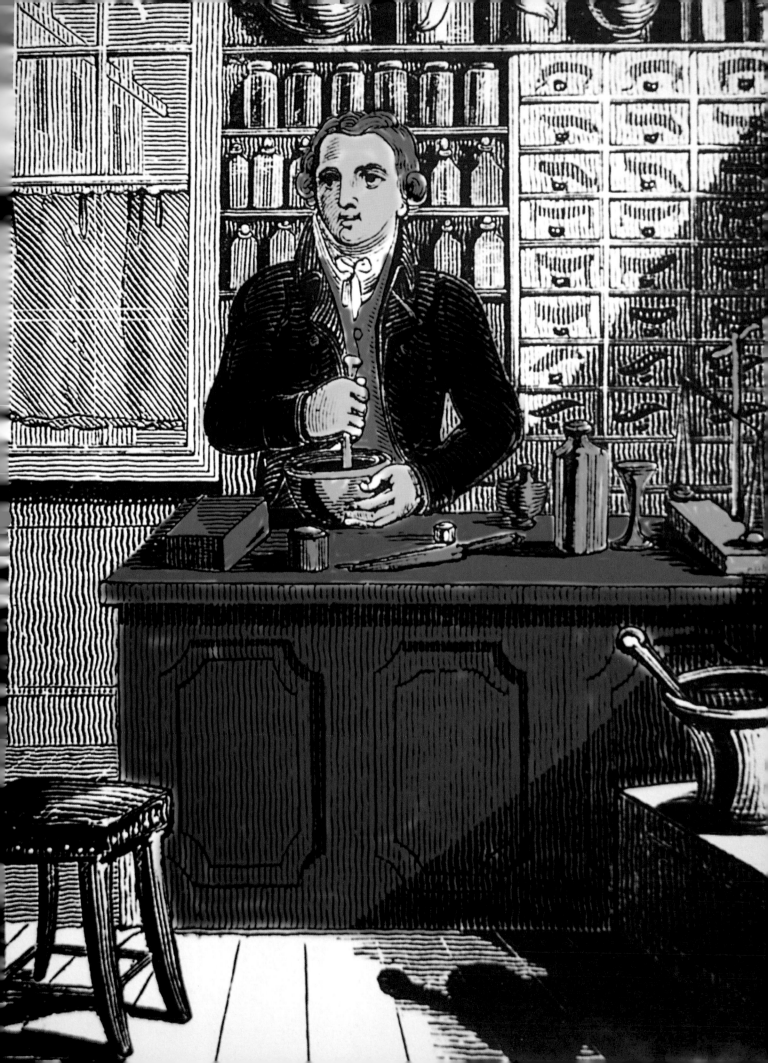

► *Benjamin Rush mixed new ideas about care for people with mental illness with old-fashioned ideas such as bleeding patients.*

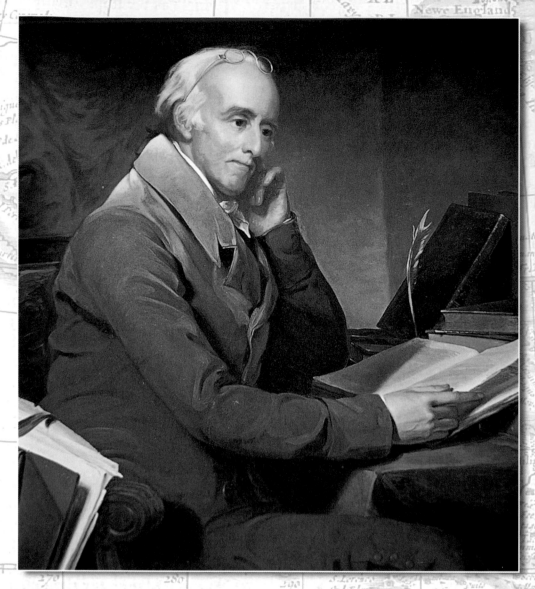

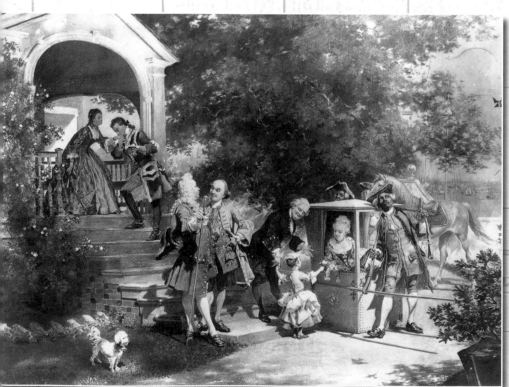

◄ *By the time Benjamin Rush became a doctor, physicians had a high position in colonial society. They belonged to the upper class and enjoyed the benefits of wealth.*

Benjamin Rush

Benjamin Rush was one of the most famous doctors in colonial America. He had such a high position in society that he became one of the founders who helped create the United States.

The first doctors in the colonies were often barbers who also knew a little medicine. By the time Benjamin was born in 1746, doctors were more important. There were still no real medical schools in America, however. Rush went to study at the university in Edinburgh, Scotland.

In 1769, when Rush returned to Philadelphia, Pennsylvania, he became a professor at the first medical school in America. He had new ideas about looking after people with **mental illness**. He said it was important to treat them kindly. He is still called the father of American **psychiatry**.

Rush became famous in 1793, when yellow fever killed 4,000 people in Philadelphia. Rush used new cures to save many of the sick. He also cut them to let their blood run out, which other doctors thought was old fashioned.

Beyond Colonial Medicine

By the time the colonies joined together as the United States in 1776, medicine was well established in America. There were medical schools in New York City and Philadelphia, so doctors could train in America. Many doctors understood better how to avoid disease. They taught their patients about the importance of a good diet, regular exercise, and cleanliness. Most doctors were giving up practices like using leeches to suck out the blood.

There were more drugs that helped clean out the body. The colonists had learned some cures from their Native American neighbors, and they had learned how to make cures from plants that the first European settlers had not recognized.

The work of doctors like Benjamin Rush led to better care for people with mental illness. They had once been ignored, but were now treated more kindly. However, the causes of mental and many other diseases were still a mystery. American doctors had much to learn.

Glossary

colonies (KAH-luh-neez) New places where people live, but where they are still ruled by their old county's leaders.

diseases (diz-EE-ziz) Sicknesses that affect living things.

dissolved (DIS-olfed) A solid mixed into a liquid.

germs (JERMZ) Tiny living things that can cause sickness and infection.

immunity (i-MYOO-ne-tee) Protection against catching a disease.

infected (in-FEKT-ed) Having caught a disease.

inoculation (ih-nah-kyoo-LAY-shun) A way to prevent disease by putting a tiny amount of the disease into someone's body using a needle.

leeches (LEECH-ez) Wormlike animals that live in water.

lice (LYCE) Small creatures that live on other creatures and people.

malaria (mal-AIR-nee-uh) A disease transferred by mosquito bites.

mental illness (MEN-tul IL-nes) A sickness that affects the mind.

merchants (MER-chunz) People who bought and sold goods.

midwives (MID-whyvs) People trained to help women give birth.

plantations (plan-TAY-shunz) Very large farms where crops like tobacco were grown.

psychiatry (SY-ky-uh-tree) The study of problems of the mind.

scurvy (SCUR-vee) A disease caused by a lack of Vitamin C.

shaman (SHAH-muhn) A priest in some religions who uses magic to heal the sick and to control events in people's lives.

sweat baths (SWET baths) A way Native Americans got rid of impurities.

vermin (VER-min) Animals that harm crops, houses, or food, such as mice, rats, or fleas.

Index

A
apothecary, 18

B
bleeding, 17, 21

C
colonies, 5–6, 21
crops, 5, 6

D
doctors, 5, 14, 17, 21–22

F
Florida, 9

G
germs, 5, 9, 13, 14

I
immunity, 9
inoculation, 13

L
leeches, 17, 22

M
medical schools, 21
midwives, 14

N
Native Americans, 5–6, 9–10, 13, 22

P
Philadelphia, Pennsylvania, 21–22

R
Rush, Benjamin, 21, 22

S
shaman, 10
slaves, 6
smallpox, 9, 13

V
Virginia, 6, 9

Primary Sources

Page 4 (top right). Portrait of Louis XIV, painted in 1701 by Hyacinthe Rigaud. The picture is held at the Louvre, Paris. **Page 4 (center left).** Poster printed in London, 1609. **Page 4 (bottom).** Map of Roanoke drawn by John White in 1585. **Page 7 (top).** *The arrival of Englishmen in Virginia.* Thomas Harriet published this map in *A Briefe and True Report of the New Found Land of Virginia* in 1590 **Page 8 (bottom).** Jacques Cartier Landing in Canada; detail from the Vallard Chart, drawn on vellum by an anonymous artist around 1547. **Page 11 (top).** Carving of a Native American shaman and two helping spirits, wood carving, no dates. **Page 11 (bottom left).** Eagle medicine bundle, no details. **Page 11 (bottom right).** Member of the Assiniboine people emerging from a ceremonial sweatbath, photograph, no date. **Page 12 (top).** *Cotton Mather.* This engraving is based on a 1728 engraving by Peter Pelham held at the American Antiquarian Society and at Yale University Art Gallery. **Page 12 (center right).** This poster for slave sale dates from around the 1780s. It is held at the Library of Congress Prints and Photographs Division. **Page 12 (bottom).** This drawing was made by Charles Lawrence in 1930. It is based on the original plans from 1657. **Page 15 (top).** Engraving of an amputation from surgical manual printed in 1739. **Page 16 (top left).** Surgeon's insterment case, instruments with tortoiseshell handles, seventeenth century. **Page 16 (top right).** The label in the lid of the medicine chest is a guarantee by a member of the Washington family that the chest belonged to George Washington at his home, Mount Vernon. It was passed down through the family. **Page 16 (bottom).** The holes in the lids of these jars allowed the leeches to breathe. Look up the practice of using leeches to find out the dates between which such jars might have been used. **Page 19.** Apothecary's shop, eighteenth-century engraving. **Page 20 (bottom).** Portrait of Benjamin Rush. Based on a painting by Thomas Sully.

Web Sites

Due to the changing nature of Internet links, PowerKids Press has developed an online list of Web sites related to the subject of this book. This site is updated regularly. Please use this link to access the list: www.powerkidslinks.com/pselca/mca.